Published By Adam Gilbin

@ Larry Johnson

Crock Pot: Quick and Easy Crock Pot Recipes for

Vibrant Health and Weight Loss

All Right RESERVED

ISBN 978-1-990666-85-8

I0554707

TABLE OF CONTENTS

Cauliflower And Ham Breakfast Casserole

Ingredients:

- Ground pepper, to taste.

- 1 Cauliflower head, shredded.

- 2 small onion, diced.

- 2 chopped green onion.

- 2 cup of cubed ham, grass-fed.

- Half a cup of bacon, grass-fed.

- 1 ½ Cups of egg whites.

- 1/2 Cup of raw milk or full-fat cream.

- 1 Teaspoon of powdered mustard.

- 1 Teaspoon Himalayan salt.

Directions:

1. Grease the inside of the Crock-Pot with the Keto-approved oil of your choice.
2. Beat the egg whites, milk or cream, mustard, salt and pepper.
3. Layer the bottom with shredded cauliflower, onion, and ham (only use 1/3 of each ingredient). Pour 1/3 of the egg whites over the top.
4. Repeat step three twice more.
5. Take your egg white mix and pour it over the Ingredients: in the crock pot.
6. Leave for 5-6 hours on low.
7. When d2, top with chopped green onion. Serve.

Asparagus Breakfast Casserole

Ingredients:

- 1 1/2 cups of full-fat cream or raw milk

- 1 1/4 teaspoons of salt

- ½ teaspoon of Himalayan pink salt

- ½ teaspoon of pepper

- 2 of cups of shredded, low-lactose cheddar cheese

- 1 half cup of ghee or coconut oil

- 10 strips of bacon

- 2 bunches of asparagus

- 1 ½ cups of fresh Roma tomatoes

- 1 bunch of green onions, chopped

- 8 ounces of chevre or semi-soft goat cheese

- 8 eggs

Directions:

1. Grease the Crock-Pot with your favorite Keto-friendly cooking oil.
2. Layer bacon, asparagus, onions, cheese, chevre, and Roma tomato slices on the bottom.
3. Alternate layers, so you should have 2-3 separate layers of vegetables.
4. Whisk eggs, salt pepper, and butter together. pour mixture over layers of vegetables.
5. Cover and cook 5-6 hours, or until eggs are cooked thoroughly, on low.
6. When d2, serve. Top with chopped green onion or chives.

Slow Cooker Moroccan Chicken

Ingredients:

- 1 tsp turmeric powder

- 1/2 tsp coriander powder

- 1 tsp cinnamon powder

- 1/2 tsp cardamom powder

- Optional: 1/4 - 1/2 tsp cayenne powder

- 4 cloves of fresh garlic, minced

- 1 and 1/2 TBS fresh grated ginger

- 1 and 1/2 tsp unrefined sea salt

- 2 cups homemade b2 broth

- 2-3 pounds chicken thighs and drumsticks (I used 4 and 4)

- 1 TBS ghee or coconut oil

- 1/2 of a medium onion, sliced into half rounds

- 1 tsp cumin powder

- 1 cup dried apricots, roughly chopped

- 2 cups sweet potatoes (or carrots or winter squash), cubed into bite-sized pieces

Directions:

1. Combine cumin, turmeric, coriander, cinnamon, cardamom, and minced garlic (and optional cayenne) in a small bowl. Set aside.
2. Melt the fat of choice on medium heat in a large skillet and cook chicken pieces for 3 minutes on each side.
3. You may need to do this in batches if your pan is not big enough.
4. Transfer into crock pot as you are d2.
5. When chicken is d2, add onions to pan and saute for 3-4 minutes.

6

6. Add spice mixture and saute another 30 seconds to bring out the flavors.

7. Add extra fat if it begins to stick. Turn off heat.

8. Add b2 broth, ginger, and sea salt into skillet and then pour entire mixture mixture over the chicken in the crock pot.

9. Cook for 3 hours on LOW then add the dried apricots and chopped sweet potatoes (or carrots/winter squash). Cook for at least another 3 hours.

Paleo Spicy Rib Appetizer

Ingredients:

- 2 tsp cayenne

- 1 tsp sweet basil, dried

- 1 tsp cumin

- 3 lbs pork spare ribs

- 2 tbsp paprika

- 1 tsp chili powder

- Salt and pepper to taste after dish is cooked

For the sauce

- 3 cloves garlic, crushed

- 1/2 small onion, minced

- 1 tbsp fresh lime juice

- 2 pinches of salt

- 1 cup tomatoes, peeled and chopped

- 2 serrano peppers, chopped and peeled

- 2 tbsp apple cider vinegar

Directions:

1. Cut ribs into single pieces.
2. Rub pieces with the spices and place in the slow cooker.
3. Put tomatoes in a bowl, smash them with a fork and mix in the rest of the sauce Ingredients:.
4. Pour mixture over the ribs, cover and cook on low for 4 to 6 hours until ribs are tender.

Slow Cooker Corn Chowder

Ingredients:

- 3/4 teaspoon dried thyme, crushed

- 1/8 teaspoon paprika

- 4 cups frozen whole kernel corn

- 2 cups milk

- 3 tablespoons cornstarch

- 2 tablespoons dry white wine

- 1 tablespoon snipped fresh thyme

- 4 slices bacon, crisp-cooked, drained, and crumbled

- 1 tablespoon vegetable oil

- 1 cup finely chopped carrots (2 medium)

- 1/2 cup finely chopped celery (1 stalk)

- 1/3 cup finely chopped onion (1 small)

- 3 cups peeled and cubed russet potatoes (about 1 pound)

- 3 cups reduced-sodium chicken broth

- 1 bay leaf

- 3/4 teaspoon salt

- Cracked black pepper

Directions:

1. In a medium saucepan heat oil over medium-high heat.
2. Add carrots, celery, and onion; cook about 7 minutes or until vegetables are tender, stirring occasionally.
3. Transfer mixture to a 4- to 6-quart slow cooker.

4. Stir in potatoes, broth, bay leaf, salt, dried thyme, and paprika.

5. Cover and cook on low-heat setting about 3 hours or on high-heat setting about 1-1/2 hours or until potatoes are tender.

6. Stir in corn and milk. Cover and cook about 1 hour or until heated through.

7. In a small bowl stir together cornstarch and wine; stir into mixture in cooker. Cover and cook for 10 minutes more. Stir in fresh thyme.

8. Using a potato masher, gently mash potatoes until soup is slightly thickened.

9. Sprinkle each serving with crumbled bacon and cracked pepper.

Moist & Tender Turkey Breast

Ingredients:

- 1 tablespoon brown sugar

- 1/2 teaspoon coarsely ground pepper

- 1/4 teaspoon salt

- 1 b2-in turkey breast (6 to 7 pounds)

- 4 fresh rosemary sprigs

- 4 garlic cloves, peeled

- 1/2 cup water

Directions:

1. Place turkey breast, rosemary, garlic and water in a 6-qt. slow cooker.
2. Mix brown sugar, pepper and salt; sprinkle over turkey.

13

3. Cook, covered, on low 4-6 hours or until
    turkey is tender and a thermometer inserted
    in turkey reads at least 170°. Yield: 12
    servings.

Slow Cooker Garlic Parmesan Chicken Wings Recipe

Ingredients:

- 1/2 cup Butter (melted)

- 6 cloves Garlic (minced)

- 1 cup Parmesan cheese (shredded)

- Green onions (or chives; optional; sliced thinly for garnish)

- 4 lb Chicken wings (separated into flats and drumettes)

- 1 tsp Sea salt

- 1/4 tsp Black pepper

Directions:

1. Get RECIPE TIPS in the post above, nutrition info + recipe notes below!

15

2. Click on the times in the Directions: below to start a kitchen timer while you cook.

3. Place the chicken wings in the bottom of a slow cooker. Season with sea salt and black pepper.

4. In a small bowl or saucepan, stir together the melted butter and minced garlic. You can melt it on the stove or in the microwave. If melting on the stove, saute the garlic for about a minute before removing from heat.

5. Pour the garlic butter mixture evenly over the chicken wings. Stir to coat.

6. Cook the wings in the slow cooker on High for 3 hours.

7. Toward the end, preheat the oven to Broil. Line a sheet pan with aluminum foil and grease well. (Wings will probably stick anyway, but it helps.)

8. Arrange the chicken wings in a single layer on the pan. Broil for about 5 minutes on each side, until crispy and golden.

9. Remove the garlic chicken wings from the oven. Top with shredded parmesan cheese.

10. Return to the oven for 1-2 minutes, until melted.

11. Garnish with green onions or chives, if desired.

Crock Pot Picadillo

Ingredients:

- 1/4 cup alcaparrado, Manzanilla olives, pimientos, capers or green olives

- 1 1/2 tsp ground cumin

- 1/4 tsp garlic powder

- 2 bay leaves

- Kosher salt and fresh pepper, to taste

- 2 1/2 lbs 93% lean ground beef

- 1 cup minced onion

- 1 cup diced red bell peppers

- 3 cloves garlic, minced

- 1/4 cup minced cilantro

- 1 small tomato, diced

- 8 oz can tomato sauce

Directions:

1. Brown meat in a large deep skillet on medium-high heat; season with generously with salt and a little pepper.
2. Use a wooden spoon to break the meat up into small pieces.
3. When meat is no longer pink, drain all the liquid from pan.
4. Add the onions, garlic and bell peppers to the meat and cook an addition 3-4 minutes.
5. Transfer the meat to the slow cooker, then add tomato, cilantro, tomato sauce, 1 1/4 cups water, alcaparrado (or olives) [I usually add some of the brine from the jar for added flavor] then add the spices.
6. Set slow cooker to HIGH for 3 to 4 hours or LOW for 6 to 8.

7. After it's ready, taste for salt and add more as needed [I added a little more cumin and garlic powder at the end as well since the crock pot tends to mute the flavors of herbs and spices].

8. Discard the bay leaves and serve over brown rice.

9. Makes about 5 3/4 cups.

Swiss Steak

Ingredients:

- 1/2 celery rib, cut into 1/2—inch slices

- 1/2 1]) beef round steak, cut into six pieces

- 1 1/ 2 cans (8 oz) tomato sauce

- 2/ 3 tbsp all—purpose flour

Directions:

1. Combine flour, some salt and pepper to taste in a resalable plastic bag.

2. Add the steak to the bag. Seal and shake to Coat.

3. Place onions in a crock-pot. Put the coated chops, celery and tomato sauce on top.

4. Cover and cook for 8 bolus on low.

Pork Chops With Rubbed Spices

Ingredients:

- 1/4 tbsp curry powder, dried

- 1/4 tbsp ground cumin

- 1/2 lb pork chops

- 1/4 tbsp rosemary, dried

- 1/4 tbsp thyme, dried

Directions:

1. Prepare seasonings: rosemary, thyme, curry powder, cumin, and salt and pepper to taste.
2. Evenly coat the chops with the seasoning mixture
3. Add some oil in the crock-pot before adding the coated meat.
4. Cover and cook for 4 hours on high, 6 hauls on medium, or 8 hauls on low

Egg Casserole With Sausage And Cheese

Ingredients:

- 3 1/4 tablespoons sliced green onions 2 1/2 teaspoons onions for garnish

- 12 3/4 tablespoons grated cheddar cheese

- 1 green pepper, diced

- 9.6 oz. breakfast sausage links

- 5-6 eggs, beaten until well-combined Black pepper, fresh ground

- 1 teaspoons Spike Seasoning

- 9 1/2 tablespoons cottage cheese, rinsed and drained 1 1/4 teaspoons, divided

Directions:

1. Grease a crockpot with non-stick spray or olive oil. Then place cottage cheese into a fine

mesh colander. Put the cheese in the sink and rinse with water to wash away the creamy part.

2. In a frying pan, heat a teaspoon of olive oil over medium high heat and cook half of the sausage links until fully browned. Transfer the sausage onto a cutting board to cool down.

3. Now heat a teaspoon of oil and cool the remaining half of the sausage and move it to the cutting board too. You can cook the sausages together if your pan can accommodate them.

4. Heat a teaspoon of oil and brown the pepper pieces for about 2 or 3 minutes. You can cook them directly if you want them somehow crunchy.

5. Once d2, cut the sausage links into halves and layer them in the crockpot along with diced or stripped green peppers.

6. Season with cottage cheese and then with the grated cheddar cheese.

7. Top the mixture with sliced onions and top with black pepper and spike seasoning.

8. At this point, beat the eggs until well incorporated and then pour over the cut sausages, cheese and cottage cheese.

9. Distribute the peppers and sausages in the cooking pot using a fork.

10. Close the lid in place and cook the mixture on low heat for 2 hours or more until the cheese is well melted and the eggs are firm in the center.

11. Finally, top with sliced green onions and enjoy the breakfast hot!

Turkey Crusted Crockpot Breakfast

Ingredients:

- 1/4 teaspoons Mrs. Dash

- 1/4 teaspoons fennel seed

- 1/4 teaspoons sage

- 1/4 teaspoons onion powder

- 1/4 teaspoons garlic powder

- 0.5 pound lean ground turkey

- 12 tablespoons shredded Monterey Jack cheese

- 1/4 teaspoons pepper

- 1/2 cup cottage cheese

- 3 eggs

- 1/2 chopped red bell pepper

- 1/4 chopped onion

Directions:

1. Put the raw turkey meat in the slow cooker and then stir in onion, garlic, fennel, sage and the Mrs. Dash. Stir the Ingredients: together to blend.

2. Spread the turkey meat over the bottom of the slow cooker using the back of the spoon.

3. Then chop the veggies and now layer them over the poultry meat.

4. In a medium-sized bowl, whisk the eggs.

5. Then stir in cottage cheese, pepper and salt into the whisked eggs and pour the cheese mixture over the veggies and turkey in the slow cooker.

6. Top the Ingredients: with shredded cheese and cook them on low until set, preferably overnight.

7. If you like it, use low fat turkey sausage as the crust.

Vegetable Soup, Chicken And Barley

Ingredients:

- .Barley 60 ml (1/4 cup), beaded

- Chicken breasts 2, skinless diced

- Cream of tomato 1 box of 284 ml, condensed

- .A mix of fresh vegetables for soup 750 ml (3 cups)

Directions:

1. In the sluggish cooker, join the vegetable stock with the tomato cream.
2. Add the vegetable blend, grain, and chicken.
3. Cover it and afterward cook for 8 to 10 hours at low intensity.

Mixed Veggies Burrito

Ingredients:

- 1 teaspoon butter

- .1 tablespoon mayonnaise

- ½ avocado, chopped

- 1 tomato, chopped

- 1 teaspoon chili flakes

- 1 teaspoon salt

- 1-pound chicken fillet, cut into strips

- 1 red bell pepper, cut into strips

- 1 zucchini, cut into strips

- 1 eggplant, cut into strips

- ½ cup coconut cream

- 4 keto tortillas

Directions:

1. In the simmering pot, blend the chicken in with the pepper and different fixings aside from the avocado, mayonnaise and tortillas.

2. Close the top and cook the elements for 8 hours on Low.

3. Spread the chicken blend on every tortilla, likewise partition the leftover fixings, roll and serve.

Hearty Chicken Soup

Ingredients:

- 1 cup wild rice

- 1 cup green beans

- 2 bay leaves

- 1 cup chopped parsley leaves

- ¼ tsp. ground black pepper

- 1½ lbs. b2less chicken breast

- 12 cups organic chicken broth

- 2 cups white onions, diced

- 4 garlic cloves, peeled and minced

- 2 cups celery, diced

- 2 cups carrots, peeled and diced

Directions:

1. Place all the Ingredients:, except for the parsley, into a crock pot.

2. Cook on a 'High' setting for 4 hours or on a 'Low' setting for 6-7 hours.

3. Remove the chicken and using two forks, shred the chicken into pieces.

4. Return the shredded chicken to the soup, top with fresh parsley, serve and enjoy.

Loso Roasted Tomato Soup

Ingredients:

- ½ tsp. extra-virgin olive oil

- 2 cups low-sodium chicken or vegetable broth

- Black pepper, to taste

- 2 lbs. Roma tomatoes, sliced

- 1 Spanish onion, coarsely chopped

- 4-6 whole garlic cloves, peeled

To garnish:

- Fresh basil

Directions:

1. Line a baking sheet with aluminum foil, and set aside.
2. Preheat the oven to 210C/425F.

3. In a single layer, lay the sliced tomatoes, flesh side facing up, whole garlic cloves, and onion on the prepared baking sheet.

4. Drizzle with olive oil and season with black pepper.

5. Roast the vegetables for 30-40 minutes or until they begin to char and caramelize but not burn.

6. Add the onions, tomatoes, and garlic to the crock pot along with the vegetable or chicken broth.

7. Stir to mix and cook on a 'High' setting for 2 hours.

8. Enjoy!

Breakfast Sausage Casserole

Ingredients:

- 1/2 cup almond milk

- 1/2 cup onion, chopped

- 1/4 cup coconut milk

- 1 red bell pepper, seeded and chopped

- 1 orange bell pepper, seeded and chopped

- 1 tsp. salt

- 1/4 tsp. black pepper

- 16 eggs

- 1 lb. white sweet potatoes, shredded

- 8 oz. breakfast sausage, chopped

- 6 oz. bacon, chopped

- Softened ghee, for greasing the crockpot

- Scallions, for garnish

Directions:

1. Put the onion, bacon and sausage in a pan and cook for about 10 minutes, till the sausage is browned. Drain the excess fat.

2. Grease the slow cooker with generously with ghee. Add the shredded sweet potatoes and press.

3. Add the meat and sprinkle chopped bell peppers.

4. In a large bowl whisk together the eggs, almond and coconut milk, salt and pepper.

5. Pour the mixture into the slow cooker.

6. Cook on low for 8 hours.

Banana Coconut Bread

Ingredients:

- 1/4 cup h2y

- 1/4 cup coconut oil

- 1/4 cup cocoa powder, raw and unsweetened

- 1/4 cup chopped walnuts

- 1 tsp. vanilla extract

- 1 tsp. baking soda

- Pinch of salt

- 5 large eggs

- 2 ripe bananas, mashed

- 1 cup coconut flour

- 1/2 cup sorghum flour

Directions:

1. Mix coconut and sorghum flour, add the baking powder and salt. Set aside

2. In another bowl mix the bananas with coconut oil, h2y, eggs and vanilla extract.

3. Now combine the dry Ingredients: with the liquid 2s. Mix well.

4. Add the chopped walnuts and mix again.

5. Grease the slow cooker with coconut oil, add the dough and cook on low for 8 hours.

6. When d2, remove from crockpot, slice into 10 pieces and serve.

Scrambled Tofu Burrito

Ingredients:

- 4 tbsp - green pepper (minced)

- 11/2 cup (350 ml) – water

- 1 tsp - turmeric (ground)

- 1/2 tsp - cumin (ground)

- 1/2 tsp - chili powder

- 1/2 tsp - smoked paprika

- 3 cups cooked or 2 cans (15 ounces) - black beans (rinsed and drained)

- 400 g - crumbled tofu

- 4 tbsp - cooked onion

- Pepper and salt to taste

- 8 - whole-wheat tortillas (use gluten-free)

Directions:

1. Add all Ingredients: from black beans (through smoked paprika) to pot. Cook on LOW heat for 7-9 hours.

2. Add salt and pepper as per taste. Spoon 1/4 mixture onto each tortilla. Add extra topping of choice, roll up tortillas and serve.

Brown Rice, Cheddar And Broccoli Casserole

Ingredients:

- 2 tbsp - flour

- 2 cups - milk

- 1 cup - shredded low-fat cheddar cheese (divided equally)

- 1 1/2 cups - uncooked brown rice

- 1 pound - broccoli florets (finely chopped)

- 1/4 cup - Parmesan cheese (grated)

- 2 tbsp - butter

- 1/4 cup - fresh mushrooms (finely chopped)

- 1/2 - small onion (finely chopped)

- 1 - clove garlic (minced)

- Ground black pepper and salt to taste

Optional:

- 1/2 cup - walnuts chopped

Directions:

1. Add butter to a large saucepan. When the butter melts, add onion, garlic and mushrooms.
2. Saute over medium flame until soft. Add salt and pepper.
3. Stir in flour and cook until the mixture is browned.
4. Add the milk slowly and boil. Keep stirring for 2 minute and then remove from heat.
5. Add half the cheese. Keep blending until the cheese melts.
6. Add uncooked rice, broccoli and the cheese sauce to crockpot.
7. Add water and stir once before cooking on LOW for 6 hours. Cook till rice is tender.

8. Add the remaining Cheddar and the Parmesan. Cook for another hour.

9. Sprinkle walnuts on top before you serve.

Creamy Keto "Hash Browns"

Ingredients:

- 2 Tablespoons of curry powder

- 2 Tablespoons of nutritional yeast

- 1 Tablespoon of coconut or avocado oil

- Salt and pepper to taste

- 4 Cups of cauliflower, grated into "rice"

- 1 ½ Cups water

- 1/4th Cup liquid aminos

- 2/3 Cup whole-fat sour cream or whole-fat yogurt

Directions:

1. Shred your cauliflower until you have 4 cups.

2. Depending on the size of your cauliflower, this is approximately 2 medium-sized cauliflower heads.

3. Put cauliflower shreds in Crock-Pot, followed by the water, liquid aminos, and oil.

4. Cover and cook on low for 2 hours, or until cauliflower is tender like a traditional potato hash brown.

5. Turn off heat. Mix around and add in sour cream, curry, and nutritional yeast.

6. Enjoy with a poached egg, avocado, or your favorite Keto-friendly breakfast meat.

Egg White Broccoli-Swiss Frittata

Ingredients:

- 1/4 cup of grated parmesan cheese

- 1 teaspoon of Himalayan pink salt

- Pepper to taste

- $1/4^{th}$ cup of chives

- 4 cups of broccoli florets, cut small

- 1/2 cup of full-fat cottage cheese

- ¾ cup of full-fat Swiss cheese

- 2 cups of egg whites, beaten

Directions:

1. Grease the inside of your Crock-Pot with your favorite Keto-friendly oil.

2. Rinse the cottage cheese under water, using a fine-mesh strainer, until only the curds and not the milk remain. Let curds sit in strainer in the sink or over a paper towel while you prepare the Swiss cheese and broccoli.

3. Grate the parmesan cheese and set aside.

4. Cut the broccoli into bite-sized florets and set aside.

5. Layer the bottom of the Crock-Pot with the broccoli. Top with first the cottage cheese and then the parmesan cheese.

6. Cook on low for three hours, or until the egg whites are set.

7. Chop chives and serve on top of slightly-cool frittata.

Crock Pot Pork Loin

Ingredients:

- 2 tablespoon basil, dried

- 1/4 teaspoon black pepper, freshly ground

- 1/2 teaspoon sea salt, (optional)

- 1 1/2 pound pork loin

- 1 can tomato sauce (15 oz)

- 2 medium zucchini, sliced

- 1 head cauliflower, separated into medium florets

Directions:

1. Add all of the Ingredients: to a large crock pot.
2. Cook on high for 3-4 hours or low 7-8 hours.

Slow Cooker Rotisserie Chicken

Ingredients:

- 1 tsp. sea salt

- 1 tsp. paprika

- 1 tsp. ground black pepper

- 1/2 tsp. cayenne pepper (optional)

- 1 whole chicken (4-5 lbs.), rinsed and patted dry

- 2 Tbsp. extra virgin olive oil

- 1 tsp. dried thyme

- 1 tsp. garlic powder

Directions:

1. Make about 6 balls of aluminum foil and line the bottom of your slow cooker with them

(you don't have to crunch the balls up too tight).

2. You can also substitute chopped vegetables such as onion, carrots and celery if you don't want to use aluminum foil, or get 2 of these handy slow-cooker roasting racks that helps keep items elevated while cooking.

3. Combine the thyme, garlic powder, paprika, salt and pepper in a small bowl.

4. Rub the oil all over the chicken, then and rub the seasoning over, making sure the chicken is evenly coated.

5. Place chicken in the crock pot on top of the chopped vegetables.

6. Cook on low for 6-8 hours or until chicken is cooked through.

7. As an optional finishing step, place the oven rack in the bottom third of the oven and turn the oven on to broil.

8. Carefully place the chicken in a baking dish and allow to broil for about 5-10 minutes until the skin is crispy and brown.

Slow Cooker Butter Chicken

Ingredients:

- 2 Tbsp Arrowroot Flour

- 2 tsp Garam Masala

- 1 tsp Curry Powder

- 1/2 tsp ground Ginger

- 1/2 tsp Chili Powder, Add more if you like it hotter

- 1 pinch Sea Salt

- 1 pinch Black Pepper

- 1 Tbsp Organic Coconut Oil

- 3 - 4 whole Garlic, crushed

- 1 whole Onion, diced

- 1 3/4 cup Coconut Milk

- 3/4 cup Tomato Paste

- 2 1/5 lb Skinless Chicken Breast

Directions:

1. Heat coconut oil in a large saucepan on medium high heat.
2. Add onion and garlic, cook, stirring frequently for approximately 3 minutes or until the onions have become translucent.
3. Add coconut milk, tomato paste, tapioca flour, garam masala, curry powder, ginger powder, chili powder and ginger powder, stirring until well combined and the sauce has started to thicken.
4. Season with salt and pepper.
5. Add chicken to the slow cooker, then add the sauce and mix through the chicken.
6. Cover and cook on low heat for 5 hours.
7. Cover and cook on low heat for 5 hours.

8. Serve with coriander and your favorite side.

Gingerbread Pudding Cake

Ingredients:

- 3/4 teaspoon baking soda

- 1/4 teaspoon salt

- 1/2 teaspoon ground cinnamon

- 1/2 teaspoon ground ginger

- 1/4 teaspoon ground allspice

- 1/8 teaspoon ground nutmeg

- 1/2 cup chopped pecans

- 6 tablespoons brown sugar

- 3/4 cup hot water

- 2/3 cup butter, melted

- 1/2 cup molasses

- 1 cup water

- 1/4 cup butter, softened

- 1/4 cup sugar

- 1 large egg white

- 1 teaspoon vanilla extract

- 1-1/4 cups all-purpose flour

- Sweetened whipped cream, optional

Directions:

1. Mix molasses and 1 cup water.

2. In a bowl, cream softened butter and sugar until light and fluffy; beat in egg white and vanilla. In another bowl, whisk together flour, baking soda, salt and spices; add to creamed mixture alternately with molasses mixture, beating well after each addition. Fold in pecans.

3. Pour into a greased 3-qt. slow cooker. Sprinkle with brown sugar.

4. Mix hot water and melted butter; pour over batter (do not stir).

5. Cook, covered, on high until a toothpick inserted in center comes out clean, 2 to 2-1/2 hours.

6. Turn off slow cooker; let stand 15 minutes. If desired, serve with whipped cream. Yield: 8 servings.

Green Bean Casserole

Ingredients:

- 1 cup 2% milk

- 6 bacon strips, cooked and crumbled

- 1 teaspoon pepper

- 1/8 teaspoon paprika

- 4 ounces process cheese (Velveeta), cubed

- 1 can (2.8 ounces) French-fried onions

- 2 packages (16 ounces each) frozen cut green beans, thawed

- 2 cans (10-3/4 ounces each) condensed cream of mushroom soup, undiluted

- 1 can (8 ounces) sliced water chestnuts, drained

Directions:

1. In a 4-qt. slow cooker, combine the green beans, soup, water chestnuts, milk, bacon, pepper and paprika.

2. Cover and cook on low for 5-6 hours or until beans are tender; stir in cheese.

3. Cover and cook for 30 minutes or until cheese is melted.

4. Sprinkle with onions. Yield: 10 servings.

Crock Pot Sugar Free Bbq Pulled Chicken

Ingredients:

- 1/2 cup water

- 1/4 cup apple cider vinegar

- 1 cup sugar free ketchup use my recipe from cookbook if you have it

- 1 teaspoon maple extract

- 1/4 teaspoon cumin

- 1/4 teaspoon salt

- 1 tablespoon cocoa powder unsweetened

- 1/2 teaspoon clear liquid stevia

- 3 pounds b2less skinless chicken thighs

- 1 teaspoon smoked paprika

- 1 teaspoon onion powder

- 1 teaspoon cumin

- 1/2 teaspoon salt

- 1/4 teaspoon pepper

Directions:

1. Place the chicken on a baking sheet.
2. Whisk the paprika, onion powder, cumin, salt and pepper together.
3. Rub the dry seasonings onto the chicken on both sides. Set aside.
4. Pour the water, apple cider vinegar, and ketchup into the bottom of the crock pot.
5. Stir until combined then add the remaining Ingredients: to the crock pot.
6. Stir well then add the chicken thighs to the crock pot.
7. Cover and cook on high 4 hours or low 8 hours.

8. Uncover when finished cooking and shred thighs with 2 forks.
9. Enjoy over coleslaw or in a low carb tortilla as a burrito.

Keto Low Carb Chili Recipe - Crock Pot Or Instant Pot

Ingredients:

- 2 tbsp Worcestershire sauce

- 1/4 cup Chili powder

- 2 tbsp Cumin

- 1 tbsp Dried oregano

- 2 tsp Sea salt

- 1 tsp Black pepper

- 1 medium Bay leaf (optional)

- 2 1/2 lb Ground beef

- 1/2 large Onion (chopped)

- 8 cloves Garlic (minced)

- 2 15-oz can Diced tomatoes (with liquid)

- 1 6-oz can Tomato paste

- 1 4-oz can Green chiles (with liquid)

Directions:

1. In a skillet over medium-high heat, cook the chopped onion for 5-7 minutes, until translucent (or increase the time to about 20 minutes if you like them caramelized).

2. Add the garlic and cook for a minute or less, until fragrant.

3. Add the ground beef. Cook for 8-10 minutes, breaking apart with a spatula, until browned.

4. Transfer the ground beef mixture into a slow cooker.

5. Add remaining ingredients, except bay leaf, and stir until combined. Place the bay leaf into the middle, if using.

6. Cook for 6-8 hours on low or 3-4 hours on high. If you used a bay leaf, remove it before serving.

7. Select the "Sauté" setting on the pressure cooker (this part is done without the lid).

8. Add the chopped onion and cook for 5-7 minutes, until translucent (or increase the time to about 20 minutes if you like them caramelized).

9. Add the garlic and cook for a minute or less, until fragrant.

10. Add the ground beef. Cook for 8-10 minutes, breaking apart with a spatula, until browned.

11. Add remaining ingredients, except bay leaf, to the Instant Pot and stir until combined. (For the Instant Pot version, it is recommended to also add a cup of water or broth.) Place the bay leaf into the middle, if using.

12. Close the lid. Press "Keep Warm/Cancel" to stop the saute cycle.

13. Select the "Meat/Stew" setting (35 minutes) to start pressure cooking.

14. Wait for the natural release if you can, or turn the valve to "vent" for quick release if you're short on time.

15. If you used a bay leaf, remove it before serving.

Lamb With Mint And Green Beans

Ingredients:

- 1/8 cup freshly chopped mint leaves

- 3 cups green beans, trimmed

- 1/2 lamb leg (b2 in)

- 1 tbsp ghee, tallow or lard

Directions:

1. Pat the lamb dry with paper towels and season it with salt and pepper
2. Grease the crock—pot with ghee, tallow or lard, then put the lamb inside
3. Sprinkle with garlic and mint all over. If it makes you more comfortable, add up to half a cup of water.
4. Cover and cook for 4 hours on high.

5. Transfer the lamb to a plate, then place the green beans on the bottom of the crock—pot. Add the lamb again inside.

6. Cover and cook for another two hours on high.

Braised Lamb Stew

Ingredients:

- 1/2 cup white wine

- 1 1/2 carrots, chopped

- 1 tbsp butter

- 1 lb leg of lamb

- 1/2 cup b2 broth

Directions:

1. Rub lamb with salt, pepper and 01L Brown it in a crock—pot set on high

2. Set it aside and throw in your veggies in the crock—pot, including onion and garlic to taste.

3. When the veggies have acquired desired

4. Crispness, add in the b2 broth and white Mix thoroughly

5. Submerge the lamb legs into the mixture.

6. Cover and cook for four hours on high.

Overnight Breakfast Casserole

Ingredients:

- 1 red bell pepper, seeded and diced

- 0.4 pound rutabagas, peeled and shredded

- 3 1⁄4 tablespoons yellow onion, diced

- 2.4 ounces bacon, chopped

- 3.4 ounce bulk breakfast sausage, crumbled

- Softened ghee, to greasing the crockpot

- Dash teaspoon cracked black pepper Dash
  teaspoon dry mustard
  1/2 teaspoon sea salt
  2 tablespoons full-fat coconut milk 3 1⁄4
  tablespoons almond milk

- 6-7 large eggs, beaten
  1 orange bell pepper, seeded and diced

- Green onions, for garnish

Directions:

1. First grease the bottom and sides of a crockpot using softened ghee or palm shortening.

2. Then cook the onion, bacon and the sausage in the slow cooker until the onion is softened and the sausage browned, or for about 10 to 12 minutes.

3. Discard any excess fat. Now add in shredded rutabaga in the crockpot and press them down gently.

4. Add in the onion and meat mixture and bell peppers on top.

5. In a separate bowl, whisk together eggs, mustard, salt, milk and pepper. Pour into the crockpot.

6. Cook the mixture on low for 6 to 8 hours or until cooked through.

Crock Pot Mexican Breakfast Casserole

Ingredients:

- 1/8 teaspoon coriander

- 1/8 teaspoon garlic powder

- 2.4 ounces J2s Dairy Farm Pork Sausage Roll

- Avocado salsa, sour cream and cilantro: optional

- 1⁄4 cup Pepper Jack cheese 1⁄4 cup coconut milk
  4 eggs
  1⁄4 cup salsa

- Dash teaspoon pepper Dash teaspoon salt
  1/2 teaspoon chili powder 1/2 teaspoon cumin

Directions:

1. First cook the pork sausage in a large skillet over medium heat until it's no longer pink.

2. Season and add salsa then set aside to slightly cool down.

3. In a separate bowl, whisk the coconut milk with eggs then add in pork to the eggs.

4. Now add in Jack cheese and stir to blend. Grease the bottom of a slow cooker and pour in the egg mixture.

5. Finally cook on low for 5 hours or high for 2 1/2 hours. Serve topped with preferred toppings.

Artichoke And Asparagus Mix

Ingredients:

- ¼ teaspoon salt

- 3 eggs, beaten

- 3 tablespoons cream cheese

- ¼ cup fresh parsley

- ½ cup coconut cream

- 1 cup artichoke hearts, chopped

- 1 tablespoon butter, softened

- 1 cup asparagus, chopped

- 1 teaspoon oregano, dried

Directions:

1. In the sluggish cooker, blend the artichokes in with the asparagus and different fixings and stir.

2. Close the top and cook quiche for 3 and ½ hours on High.

Onion Soup From The Slow Cooker

Ingredients:

- Salt, pepper

- 8 slices of toasted bread

- 150 grams of cheese, grated

- 1/2 bunch of parsley, chopped

- 3 tbsp. Olive oil

- 500 ml of beef stock

- 500 ml of water

Directions:

1. Skin onions, cut into quarters and cut into rings that are not excessively thick. In giving the sluggish cooker, shower with the olive oil and blend well.

2. Cook for eight hours at high, mixing once or twice.

3. Cook the cooked onions (they will be brown, delicate and extremely sweet-smelling) with the base and the water and add season with salt and pepper.

4. Let it heat up for another 30 - an hour on HIGH.

5. Sprinkle toast with cheddar, place on a baking plate, and brown under the broiler barbecue.

6. Fill the soup into cups and put on bread; let it stew momentarily so the bread retains some broth.

7. Sprinkle with parsley and serve.

Crock Pot Lentil Soup

Ingredients:

- 1 medium carrot, diced

- 1 tbsp. extra-virgin olive oil

- 1 tsp. tomato paste

- ½ tsp. ground coriander

- ½ tsp. ground cumin

- ¼ tsp. smoked paprika

- 2 tsp. red wine vinegar

- 1 bay leaf

- 1 tsp. kosher salt

- 4 cups or 1 quart low-sodium vegetable broth

- 1 cup green lentils

- 1 14-oz. can diced tomatoes, juice and all

- 1 small yellow onion, diced

- 2 cloves garlic, minced

- 1 medium celery stalk, diced

To serve:

- Plain yogurt, extra-virgin olive oil, chopped fresh parsley or cilantro leaves

Directions:

1. Place all the Ingredients:, except the vinegar into a 4-quart crock pot. Stir well to combine.
2. Cover and cook on a 'Low' setting for 8 hours until the lentils are fork-tender.
3. Remove and discard the bay leaf and stir in the red wine vinegar.
4. Ladle the soup into bowls and top with yogurt, extra-virgin olive oil and chopped fresh parsley or cilantro.

Hearty Crock Pot Minestr2 Soup

Ingredients:

- 1 15-oz. can red kidney beans, drained and rinsed

- 1 28-oz. can diced tomatoes, with all the juice

- 4 cups no-fat vegetable stock or broth

- 2 cups water

- 2 tbsp. vegetable stock base

- Parmesan rind, or 1-inch chunk Parmesan

- 2 tbsp. tomato paste

- 1¼ tbsp. dried Italian seasoning

- ⅛ tsp. red pepper flakes

- 1½ cups yellow onion, finely diced

- 2-3 tbsp. garlic, minced

- 1 cup celery, finely sliced

- 1 cup carrots, peeled and finely diced

- 1 15-oz. can cannellini beans, drained and rinsed

- 2 bay leaves

To Add 20-25 Minutes before Serving:

- 1½ cups dried ditalini or other small pasta

- 1 cup zucchini, finely

To Add 5 Minutes before Serving:

- 1 cup frozen green beans, cut

- 1½ cups fresh baby spinach, roughly chopped

Directions:

1. Add the first 15 Ingredients: to 6-quart crock pot.

2. Everything well and cover with the crock pot lid.

3. Cook on a 'High' setting for 3 – 4 hours or on a 'Low' setting for 6-8 hours.

4. 25 - 30 minutes before serving, add the dried pasta and diced zucchini and stir well.

5. Cover continue cooking on a 'High' setting for 20-25 minutes.

6. Then 5 minutes before serving, add in the frozen baby spinach and cut green beans and cook on a 'High' setting for 5 minutes.

7. This soup is traditionally served with grate parmesan on top. Ladle into bowls and enjoy!

Mexican Breakfast Casserole

Ingredients:

- 1 large onion, chopped

- 1 red bell pepper, chopped

- 2 Tablespoons guacamole, mild

- 1 tsp. salt

- 1/4 tsp. ground pepper

- 1/4 tsp. garlic powder

- 1/8 tsp. cumin

- 8 large eggs

- 8 slices turkey bacon

- 8 oz. (s), mushrooms, white, raw

- 1 cup sweet potato, cubed

Directions:

1. Fry the bacon until crispy. Crumble and set aside.

2. In the same pan with the bacon grease fry the onions until soften.

3. In a large bowl whisk the eggs, add the sweet potato, mushrooms, red bell pepper, fried bacon and onion. Season with salt, ground pepper, garlic powder and cumin. Stir to combine.

4. Transfer the mixture into the slow cooker.

5. Cook on low for 8 hours.

6. When d2 cut to 8 pieces, serve with guacamole.

Easy Breakfast Pie

Ingredients:

- 1 tsp. dried basil

- 1/2 tsp. garlic powder

- 1/2 tsp. salt

- 1/4 tsp. pepper

- 1 lb(s). Ground beef

- 4 oz. mushrooms chopped

- 8 large eggs, whisked

- 1 sweet potato, shredded

- 1 large onion, chopped

Directions:

1. Mix all of the Ingredients: in a large bowl.

2. Grease the slow cooker with coconut oil, to make sure that n2 of the egg sticks to it.

3. Pour the mixture. Set to low on 8 hours.

4. Slice it like a pie, and serve.

Ham & Chard Stuffed Breakfast Peppers

Ingredients:

- 1/4th cup chopped Swiss chard

- 1/4th cup grated Swiss cheese

- 1/4th cup chopped parsley

- Himalayan pink salt & pepper to taste

- 1/4th cup water

- 2 cups egg whites

- 6-8 Bell peppers, various colors

- 1 cup cubed ham

Directions:

1. Grease the inside of your Crock-Pot with your favorite Keto-friendly oil.

2. Cut the tops of the bell peppers off so that they look like cups.

3. Put equal parts ham and chard into the bell peppers.

4. Pour egg whites on top ham and chard.

5. Sprinkle Swiss cheese on top of each stuffed pepper.

6. Turn Crock-Pot to low and pour 1/4th cup of water into the pot (this helps steam the eggs). Place stuffed peppers in to follow.

7. Cook on low for 2 hours, or until eggs are set in each pepper.

8. Serve topped with parsley and with a side of your favorite Keto-approved fruit.

Roasted Red Pepper & Asparagus With Gorgonzola Cheese

Ingredients:

- 1 tablespoon of extra-virgin olive oil

- 3 tablespoons of lemon juice

- Himalayan pink salt

- Pepper to taste

- 1/3 cup of gorgonzola cheese, crumbled

- 1 cup of b2 broth or ½ cup of liquid aminos

- 2 bunches of fresh asparagus

- 2 large red bell peppers

Directions:

1. Season the inside of your Crock-Pot with your favorite Keto-friendly oil.

2. Cut bell peppers into bite-sized strips.

3. Place in crock pot with asparagus, broth or aminos, and extra-virgin olive oil.

4. Cook on low for 45 minutes, or until asparagus is chewable and soft.

5. In the Crock-Pot, season peppers and asparagus with salt, pepper, and lemon juice. Let sit with the heat off for 10 minutes.

6. Plate and crumble gorgonzola on top. Serve and enjoy!

Slow Cooker Ham

Ingredients:

- 4 tbs Coconut Oil

- Zest of 1 Orange

- 1 tbs Apple Cider Vinegar

- 1 4-6 lb Ham Roast

- 1/4 cup H2y

- 1/2 cup Orange Juice

- 2 tsp Dried Rosemary

Directions:

1. Place ham in slow cooker.
2. Put the rest of the Ingredients: on the ham.
3. Cook on low for 4-6 hours.

Slow Cooker Jalapeño Popper Chicken Chili

Ingredients:

- 2 tsp chili powder

- 2 tsp dried oregano

- 2 tsp kosher salt

- 1 tsp ground cumin

- 1/4 tsp red pepper flakes

- 1 (14 oz) can petite diced tomatoes

- 1 cup reduced sodium chicken broth

- Chopped scallions, for garnish

- 8 oz diced avocado (from 2 small haas)

- 4 oz goat cheese (optional)

- 1 medium white onion, diced

- 3 cloves minced garlic

- 1 red bell pepper, diced

- 2 jalapeños, seeds removed

- 1 large sweet potato, 14 oz

- 1 lb 93% lean ground chicken

- 1 lb 95% lean ground beef

- 2 tsp smoked paprika

Directions:

1. Place all the Ingredients: except the scallion, avocado and goat cheese in the slow cooker and cook on low 8 hours.

2. When d2, break up the ground meat with a wooden spoon and add half of the goat cheese if using.

3. Serve garnished with scallions and avocado on top.

Stuffed Peppers

Ingredients:

- 1 onion, diced

- 1 carrot, diced

- 4 cloves of garlic, minced

- 6 ounces tomato paste

- 1/4 cup homemade italian seasoning blend (equal parts marjoram, thyme, rosemary, savory, sage, oregano, basil)

- 4 bell peppers

- 1 lb ground meat

- 1/2 head of cauliflower

- Salt and pepper to taste

- 1/4 cup beef stock

Directions:

1. Pulse your cauliflower, onion, carrots, and garlic in the food processor to blend as fine as possible.

2. Do it separately if your food processor isn't large enough.

3. If you don't own 2 you can dice everything as small as possible by hand.

4. Cut the tops off of your peppers, keeping them intact and clean the seeds out.

5. Mix your vegetables in a mixing bowl with your meat, tomato paste, seasonings and salt and pepper.

6. Once all Ingredients: are combined well, spoon the mixture into your peppers and level off at the top of the pepper.

7. Place the peppers in your crock pot and put the tops of the peppers on them.

8. Pour your liquid in the bottom of the crock pot and cook on low for 6-8 hours.

Hot Mulled Ginger-Spiced Cider

Ingredients:

- 1 (1/2-inch) piece peeled fresh ginger

- 12 cups apple cider

- 1/2 cup apple jelly

- 1/4 teaspoon ground nutmeg

- 3 whole cloves

- 2 (1 x 4-inch) strips orange rind

- 2 whole allspice

- 1 (3-inch) cinnamon stick

Directions:

1. Place the first 5 Ingredients: on a 5-inch-square double layer of cheesecloth.

2. Gather edges of cheesecloth together; tie securely.

3. Place cheesecloth bag, cider, jelly, and nutmeg in an electric slow cooker.

4. Cover and cook on high for 4 hours. Remove and discard cheesecloth bag.

Grandma Dean's Chicken And Dressing

Ingredients:

- 1 medium onion, chopped

- 3 celery ribs, chopped

- 4 large eggs, lightly beaten

- 2 teaspoons ground sage

- 1/2 teaspoon pepper

- 1/4 teaspoon salt

- 1 (2 1/2-pound) rotisserie chicken, skinned, b2d, and shredded (about 4 cups)

- 6 cups coarsely crumbled cornbread

- 8 (1-ounce) firm white bread slices, torn into pieces

- 2 (14-ounce) cans chicken broth

- 2 (10 3/4-ounce) cans cream of chicken soup

- 1/2 cup butter, softened

Directions:

1. Combine first 11 Ingredients: in a large bowl.
2. Transfer mixture to a lightly greased 5-quart round slow cooker. Dot evenly with butter.
3. Cover and cook on HIGH 3 to 4 hours or on LOW 7 hours or until set. Stir well before serving.

Steamed Brown Bread With Currants And Walnuts

Ingredients:

- 1/2 teaspoon salt

- 1 cup low-fat buttermilk

- 1/3 cup molasses

- 1/2 cup dried currants

- 2 tablespoons chopped walnuts

- Vegetable cooking spray

- 1/2 cup all-purpose flour

- 1/2 cup whole-wheat flour

- 1/2 cup yellow cornmeal

- 3/4 teaspoon ground cinnamon

- 1/2 teaspoon baking soda

Directions:

1. Combine the first 6 Ingredients: in a large bowl, and make a well in center of mixture.

2. Combine buttermilk and molasses; stir well.

3. Add to flour mixture, stirring just until moistened.

4. Fold in currants and walnuts.

5. Spoon the mixture into a 13-ounce coffee can coated with cooking spray.

6. Cover with aluminum foil coated with cooking spray; secure foil with a rubber band.

7. Place the can in an electric slow cooker; add enough hot water to cooker to come halfway up sides of can.

8. Cover with lid, and cook on high-heat setting for 2 hours and 50 minutes or until a wooden pick inserted in center comes out clean. Remove can from water.

9. Let bread cool, covered, in can on a wire rack for 5 minutes.

10. Remove bread from can, and let cool completely on wire rack.

Italian Pulled Pork Ragu

Ingredients:

- 18 oz pork tenderloin

- 1 teaspoon kosher salt

- Black pepper, to taste

- 1 tsp olive oil

- 5 cloves garlic, smashed with the side of a knife

- 1 28 oz can crushed tomatoes

- 1 small jar roasted red peppers, drained (7 oz jar)

- 2 sprigs fresh thyme

- 2 bay leaves

- 1 tbsp chopped fresh parsley, divided

Directions:

1. Instant Pot: Season pork with salt and pepper.

2. Press saute button to warm, add oil and garlic and saute until golden brown, 1 to 1 1/2 minutes; remove with a slotted spoon.

3. Add pork and brown about 2 minutes on each side.

4. Add the remaining Ingredients: and garlic, reserving half of the parsley.

5. Cook high pressure 45 minutes. Natural release, remove bay leaves, shred the pork with 2 forks and top with remaining parsley.

6. Serve over your favorite pasta.

7. Slow Cooker: Season pork with salt and pepper.

8. Heat a medium skillet over medium-high heat, add oil and garlic and saute until golden brown, 1 to 1 1/2 minutes; remove with a slotted spoon.

9. Add pork and brown about 2 minutes on each side then transfer to the slow cooker with the garlic and the remaining Ingredients:, reserving half of the parsley.

10. Cook 8 hours low. Remove bay leaves, shred the pork with 2 forks and top with remaining parsley. Serve over your favorite pasta.

11. Stove Top: Season pork with salt and pepper.

12. Heat a large pot or Dutch oven over medium-high heat, add oil and garlic and saute until golden brown, 1 to 1 1/2 minutes; remove with a slotted spoon.

13. Add pork and brown about 2 minutes on each side.

14. Add the remaining ingredients to the pot including the garlic, reserving half of the parsley.

15. Bring to a boil, cook covered on low until the pork is tender, and shreds easily, about 2 hours.

16. Remove bay leaves, shred the pork with 2 forks and top with remaining parsley. Serve over your favorite pasta.

Slow Cooker Creamy Sausage And Broccoli Cheese Soup

Ingredients:

- 8 oz velveeta, cubed

- 2 cups beef stock

- 2 tbsp garlic powder

- 1 cup cheddar cheese, shredded sharp

- 8 oz breakfast sausage, browned and crumbled

- 2 cups broccoli florets

- 1 cup diced carrots

Directions:

1. In a large slow cooker, add sausage, broccoli, carrots, velveeta, beef stock, and garlic powder.

2. Cook on low 2-3 hours.

3. When soup is melted and creamy, add cheddar cheese.

4. Top with fresh cracked pepper and serve immediately.

Kerala Lamb Stew

Ingredients:

- 1 1/3 bay leaves

- 10 curry leaves

- 4 3/4 oz b2less lamb

- 1 1/3 tbsp coconut oil

- 4 1/2 oz coconut milk

Directions:

1. Marinate the mutton with the salt, pepper, chili
2. Powder and other spices desired.
3. In crock-pot, heat some coconut oil and fry the
4. Mutton browning it on each side Add bay leaves
5. Cover and cook on low for 5—6 bolus.

6. When simmering starts, add the curry leaves

7. And coconut milk Cook this for another hum:

Fall-Off-The-B2 Lamb Shanks

Ingredients:

- 2 1b lamb shanks, seas2d and browned

- 1 tbsp extra virgin olive oil

- 2 organic chicken or beef stock

- 1 tsp smoked paprika

- 2 rosemary sprigs

Directions:

1. Place lamb shanks in the crock—pot.
2. Add the chicken stock, rosemary sprigs, smoked paprika, onions, salt and pepper to taste into the crock—pot.
3. The meat should be submerged
4. Cook on high for 4 hours, or on low for 8 hours

Cauliflower Breakfast Casserole

Ingredients:

- 1/2 head cauliflower

- 1/4 teaspoon pepper

- 1/2 teaspoon Himalayan salt

- 1/8 teaspoon dry mustard

- 2 tablespoons unsweetened almond milk

- 4 large eggs

- 1 cup of shredded cheddar cheese

- 4 slices of low sodium, all natural turkey bacon, cooked and diced 1/2 small bell pepper, diced

- 1/2 small onion, diced

- Salt and pepper

113

Directions:

1. Coat a slow cooker with coconut oil or olive oil spray and set aside.

2. Then mix together dry mustard, eggs, salt, almond milk and pepper in a large bowl.

3. Put around 1/3 of the cauliflower in the bottom of the crockpot and top with 2 third of the bell pepper and onion.

4. Season with pepper and salt, and top with 2 third of the cheese and 2 third of the bacon. Repeat the layers two more rounds.

5. At this point, pour the egg mixture over the layers of the Ingredients: in the crockpot.

6. Cook until the eggs are set and browned at the top, for about 5-7 hours or so. Serve and enjoy.

Slow Cooker Cauliflower Breakfast

Ingredients:

- 1/2 leek, cut into quarter inch half-moon slices

- 6 cooked sausage links, cut into quarter inch rounds 2.5 oz. crimini mushrooms, finely diced

- 1/8 teaspoon salt

- 4 oz. Cheddar cheese

- 1/8 teaspoon salt

- 3 eggs

- 5 oz. cauliflower florets

Directions:

1. Grease a crockpot with cooking spray and set aside. Meanwhile add pieces of the

cauliflower to a heat-safe bowl along with salt.

2. Add water to the bowl and fill it to entirely cover the cauliflower, and put it in the microwave to cook for about 8 minutes.

3. As it cooks, be preparing the leeks, sausage and mushrooms. Then drain off the liquid from the half cooked cauliflower and add it to the crockpot.

4. Evenly distribute the sausage and mushrooms pieces on the cauliflower and set aside.

5. Now whisk together salt and eggs in a bowl and carefully stir in cleaned leeks. Slowly stir in half of the cheese and reserve the other half.

6. Then pour the egg mixture uniformly over the cauliflower pieces, sausage and the mushrooms.

7. Cover the Ingredients: and cook on high for about 2 to 3 hours, or until the eggs puff up.

8. At this point, sprinkle the rest of the cheese over the top and allow it to melt.

9. Then slice the casserole and enjoy. Season the dish with salt and pepper if you like.

Chili Chicken Soup

Ingredients:

- 1 t. of pepper and salt

- 1 tbsp. of each:

- Thyme

- Coconut flour

- Pepper

- Minced garlic

- .1 c. chicken stock

- 3 tbsp. lemon juice

- 3 tbsp. tomato paste

- 1 green pepper

- 2 tbsp. unsalted butter

- 8 bacon slices

- 8 chicken thighs – b2less

- ¼ c. unsweetened coconut milk

Directions:

1. Add the margarine to the sluggish cooker on the low setting. Add the thighs.
2. Thinly cut the peppers and onions and throw them into the pot.
3. Wrap the bacon over the chicken and add the seasonings.
4. Combine the wet fixings and the tomato glue.
5. Blend well and close the cover. Set the clock for six hours on low.
6. When the time is up, mix and serve.

Broccoli And Cheese Omelet

Ingredients:

- 2 tablespoons almond milk

- Salt to taste

- Pepper powder to taste

- 2 slices Swiss cheese

- 2 eggs

- 1 cup broccoli, chopped into small pieces, cooked

- Cooking spray

Directions:

1. Spray within the sluggish cooker with cooking spray.
2. Add eggs, whites, milk, salt and pepper to a bowl and whisk well.

3. Pour into the sluggish cooker.

4. Close the cover. Select 'High' and set the clock for 20-30 minutes or 'Low' and 45-an hour. Cook until the omelet is extremely delicate and set.

5. Place cheddar and broccoli at the focal point of the omelet, during the most recent 10 minutes of cooking.

6. Cook until the egg sets. Overlap the sides over the broccoli.

7. Eliminate on to a plate and serve. Cut into 2 and serve.

Crock Pot Ribollita

Ingredients:

To Cook the Beans:

- 1 head garlic, skin-on and horizontally halved

- 1 28-oz. can whole peeled Roma tomatoes in puree, chopped, with its juice

- 4 cups low-sodium chicken or vegetable broth, or plain water

- 2 tbsp. extra-virgin olive oil

- 1 lb. dried cannellini beans, rinsed and drained

- 1 – 2 sprigs fresh sage

To Cook the Vegetable Base:

- 1 cup or 2 stalks celery, chopped

- ⅔ cup chopped pancetta (optional)

- 1 tsp. dried thyme or 2 tsp. fresh thyme, snipped

- 2 tbsp. extra-virgin olive oil

- 2 cloves garlic, minced

- 1 cup or 1 large white onion, chopped

- 1 cup or 2 medium carrots, chopped

To Finish the Soup and Toast the Bread:

- 4 cups kale or Swiss chard, chopped

- ½ cup freshly grated Parmesan cheese

- 1 cup fresh parsley, snipped

- Ground black pepper, to taste

- 2 tbsp. extra-virgin olive oil

- 8 slices Italian bread like focaccia

- 1 clove garlic, for flavoring the bread

- Salt, to taste

To serve:

- Extra extra-virgin olive oil (optional)

Directions:

1. Place the cannellini beans in a large Dutch oven and add enough water to completely cover them.
2. Boil gently for 10 minutes, cover and stand for 1 hour.
3. Drain and rinse beans, then set them aside for now.
4. Fold a 100% cotton cheesecloth over on itself to form a double layer and cut out an 8-inch square.
5. Place the halved garlic head and the whole sage in center of cheesecloth. Tie closed with 100% cotton twine to form a bag.

6. In a 5 - 6-quart crock pot combine the beans, garlic-sage cheesecloth packet, tomatoes, broth, 2 tablespoons olive oil, ½ a teaspoon salt, and a ¼ teaspoon pepper.

7. Cover and cook on a 'High' setting for 5 – 6 hours or a 'Low' setting for 10 - 12 hours. The beans should be tender but not mushy.

8. Discard garlic-sage herb packet, and then using a potato masher lightly mash some of the beans, to thicken the soup and give it a creamy texture, and set aside.

9. In a large cast iron skillet heat 2 tablespoons of olive oil on medium-high.

10. Add the pancetta (if using) and cook for 3 - 5 minutes or until the pancetta has released its fat and browned.

11. Add in the onion, celery, carrots, and ½ teaspoon salt.

12. Cook for about 5 minutes or until the onion is tender. And fragrant. Stir in the minced garlic and thyme and cook about 30 seconds.

13. Set the crock pot on 'High.' Stir the sautéed vegetables into the crock pot bean mixture.

14. Cover and cook for 1 hour until the vegetables are soft and the soup has slightly thickened slightly.

15. Stir in kale and parsley* See Recipe Notes.

16. Now for the bread. Preheat the oven to 180C/350F.

17. Arrange the bread slices on a baking sheet and brush both sides with the remaining 2 tablespoons of olive oil.

18. Bake for about 10 minutes or until a light golden brown, turning once halfway through baking.

19. Cool the bread slightly and then rub the whole garlic clove over 2 side of each piece of hot toast.

20. Place 2 toast slice in each bowl.

21. Ladle the hot soup over the toast slices, and sprinkle each serving with Parmesan cheese.

22. Drizzle with additional extra-virgin olive oil and enjoy!

Fireside Beef Stew

Ingredients:

- 1 14-oz. can low-sodium beef broth

- 1 8-oz. can tomato sauce

- 2 tbsp. Worcestershire sauce

- 2 tbsp. cold water

- 4 tsp. cornstarch

- 1 tsp. mustard powder

- ¼ teaspoon ground black pepper

- 1½ lbs. b2less beef chuck roast

- 1 lb. or 2½ cups butternut squash, peeled, de-seeded, and cubed into 1-inch pieces

- 1 9-oz. packet frozen Italian green beans

- 2 small onions, cut into wedges

- 2 cloves garlic, minced

- ⅛ tsp. ground allspice

Directions:

1. Trim any excess fat from meat.

2. Cut meat into 1-inch cubes and place in a 4-quart crock pot.

3. Add in the onions, garlic and squash, and then stir in the tomato sauce and beef broth, Worcestershire sauce, dry mustard, allspice and pepper.

4. Cover and cook on a 'High' setting for 4 – 5 hours or on a 'Low' setting for 8 - 10 hours.

128

5. At this stage, if using the 'Low' setting, turn the crockpot to the 'High' setting.

6. In a small bowl, combine the cornstarch and cold water to form a cornstarch slurry.

7. Stir in the slurry and green beans into the soup and cover.

8. Cook for about 15 minutes or until sufficiently thickened. enjoy!

Breakfast Frittata

Ingredients:

- 1/4 cup white onion, chopped

- 3/4 cup spinach, cooked, chopped

- 1 tsp. sea salt

- 8 large eggs

- 4 lb. breakfast sausage

- 1/2 cup red bell pepper, chopped

- 1/2 tsp. ground pepper

Directions:

1. Mix the eggs. Add spinach, red bell pepper, onions, salt and ground pepper. Stir to combine well.

2. Grease the slow cooker with coconut oil, add the mixture. Cook on low for 3 hours.

130

Zucchini Bread

Ingredients:

- 1/3 cup coconut oil

- 2 tsp. cinnamon

- 2 tsp. vanilla extract

- 1/2 tsp. baking powder

- 1/2 tsp. baking soda

- 1/2 tsp. salt

- 3 large eggs

- 2 cups zucchini, shredded

- 1 cup almond flour

- 1/2 cup organic stevia

- 1/2 cup walnuts, chopped

- 1/3 cup coconut flour

Directions:

1. Mix almond flour, coconut flour, baking powder, baking soda, cinnamon and salt. Set aside.
2. In another bowl, whisk the eggs add coconut oil, sugar and vanilla extract. Stir until combined.
3. Combine the wet and dry Ingredients:. Add the shredded zucchini and chopped walnuts. Mix lightly to combine.
4. Pour the mixture into 8x4 silic2 bread mold.
5. Place the pan into the crockpot and cook on high 3 hours.
6. Cool completely before serving.
7. Cut into 12 pieces.

Vegetarian Fajitas

Ingredients:

- 1 medium - onion (sliced)

- 1 1/2 tsp vegetable oil (use olive oil)

- 2 tsp - cumin

- 2 tsp - chili powder

- 1/2 tsp - dried oregano

- 1/4 tsp - garlic salt

- 3 - roma tomatoes (diced)

- 4 ounce can - green chilies (diced)

- 1 large - green bell pepper (seeded and sliced)

- 1 large - red bell pepper (seeded and sliced)

- Cooking spray

Directions:

1. Spray thin coating of cooking spray on crockpot.

2. Add all Ingredients: and mix well until vegetables are coated with spices and oil.

3. Cook on LOW setting for 4 to 6 hours or on HIGH setting for 2 hours.

4. Serve with tortillas, black beans, sour cream, avocado, and any other topping of choice.

Vegetable Broth

Ingredients:

- 4 - mushrooms (chopped)

- 1 tbsp - olive oil

- 1 - bay leaf

- Few sprigs of herbs - parsley, rosemary, basil, thyme or oregano

- 10 cups - filtered water

- 1 tbsp liquid amino (use1 tbsp soy sauce or 1 tsp salt}

- 1 - large onion (chopped)

- 2 cloves - garlic (crushed)

- 3 - carrots (chopped)

- 4 stalks - celery with tops (chopped)

- 1 - bell pepper (chopped)

Directions:

1. Add the chopped vegetables and garlic to pot.
2. Drizzle olive oil on top. Add bay leaf and herbs.
3. Pour water over the vegetables and cook on LOW heat for 8 to12 hours.
4. Add liquid amino (use soy sauce or salt as alternatives). Strain liquid and cool it.
5. Serve required amount of broth and refrigerate the rest.

Garbanzo Bean And Veggie Pitas With Creamy Avocado Dressing

Ingredients:

- 3/4 tsp - salt

- 1/2 of medium sized avocado (peeled and chopped)

- 1/2 cup - plain Greek yogurt (fat-free)

- 1 tsp - red wine vinegar

- 1/2 cup - fresh basil (lightly crushed)

- 1/4 cup - fresh chives (lightly crushed)

- 2 cups - fresh spinach (chopped)

- 1 cup - grape or cherry tomatoes (halved)

- 1 cup or 8 - green onions (sliced)

- 4 - warmed pita bread rounds (halved crosswise)

- 1 1/4 cups or 8 ounces - dry garbanzo beans (chickpeas)

- 7 cups - water

- 1 - large onion (quartered)

- 4 - crushed garlic cloves

Directions:

1. Rinse the beans and drain. Place beans in crockpot.
2. Add water, onion, half of garlic cloves and salt.
3. Cover and cook on LOW setting for 8-9 hours or on High setting for 4-4 1/2 hours.
4. Cook until beans are tender. Drain and rinse the beans and let it cool.
5. Discard all solids except beans.

6. To make dressing, blend the remaining garlic, avocado, yogurt and vinegar in food processor till you get a smooth paste.

7. Add basil and chives and blend well in processor.

8. In a large bowl, combine the cooked beans, tomatoes, spinach and green onions.

9. Spoon mixture into pita breads. Add dressing on top and serve .

Greek Slow-Cook Pork Lettuce Wraps

Ingredients:

- 2 lemons, zested then juiced

- 1/3 cup of b2 broth

- 2 tablespoons of olive oil

- 1 tablespoon of oregano

- ½ teaspoon of cinnamon

- 2 sprigs of fresh mint

- 2 tablespoons of fresh-cut chives

- 2 sprigs of fresh dill

- ½ teaspoon of fennel

- 1 teaspoon of Himalayan pink salt

- 2 lbs of Pork Sirloin

- 1 tablespoon of olive oil

- 8 large iceberg lettuce leaves

- 1 chopped tomato

- Any desired, Keto-friendly toppings

- 2 tablespoons of liquid aminos

Directions:

1. Trim the pork roast of any fat and cut it into 6 pieces against the grain.

2. Heat 2 tablespoon of olive oil on medium in a separate frying pan. Brown the pork pieces on all sides.

3. Chop chives.

4. Combine broth, spices, remaining olive oil, liquid aminos, juice and zest.

5. Put browned pork in seas2d Crock-Pot.

6. Cover with the Greek-style liquid. Put fresh herbs into the pot. Cover.

7. Cook on low for 3-4 hours, or until pork comes apart with a fork.

8. Assemble desired meat into a large iceberg lettuce leaf. Roll and serve. If desired, add cheese to the roll.

www.ingramcontent.com/pod-product-compliance
Lightning Source LLC
Chambersburg PA
CBHW071002120626
46546CB00003B/898